BIAS and
BURNOUT

BIAS and
BURNOUT

10 Power Moves for
Healthcare Workplace Equity

Glennae E. Davis, RN

NaesVision
Los Angeles, California

BIAS AND BURNOUT
10 Power Moves for Healthcare Workplace Equity

Glennae E. Davis,
Bachelor of Science in Nursing, Registered Nurse

Published by NaesVision
Los Angeles, California

Editor & Designer:
Judah Freed, HokuHouse.com

Printed in the United States of America.

Softcover: ISBN: 978-0-9973495-8-0
eBook: ISBN: 978-0-9973495-9-7

This book is not intended as a substitute for the advice of a licensed or certified mental health professional. The reader is advised to consult with a trusted professional for matters relating to personal and professional health.

First edition published on July 22, 2020.

Cataloging-in-Publication Data:

Davis, Glennae, 1974 —

Bias and Burnout
10 Power Moves for Healthcare Workplace Equity

112 pages with 8 Chapters.

1. Medical / Public Health
2. Religion / Christian Living / Calling & Vocation
3. Self-Help / Self-Management / Stress Management

Dedication

For Nurses

I am continuously inspired
by your love and sacrifice, your study to heal.
Here is my best effort to save our dying profession.

*"That I may publish with the voice of thanksgiving,
and tell of all thy wondrous works."*

— Psalms 26:7

Bias and **Burnout**

Table of Contents

Acknowledgments

I wish to honor my late mother, Joan C. Davis, for being your best self. It must have been difficult living with a thought disorder while raising two girls in South Central LA. I remember the 1980s well. In spite of community and institutional challenges, you, my beloved, did an amazing job. Your reservations about the workplace and healthcare industry were correct. I recall you saying, in disillusioned laughter, your job will drive you crazy, that a doctor will medicate for seeing a piece of the truth. Mom, you never lied to me. I value the way you raised me.

To my late mentor, Raymond Earl Strain, thank you for your Godly being. With me in my early teens, you in your late thirties, a family friend, our unlikely relationship lasted and stood the test of time. You saw a difference in me, that I was worthy of being saved from gang and drug violence. An honorable and reliable man, you protected and helped shape me into the woman I am today. I am grateful for your spiritual guidance under the Nation of Islam. You would be glad to know I'm no longer living in "the dark."

To my two children, Darchell L. Sullivan and David M. Thompson, I want you both to know that you are the beat of my heart. Getting to this place of leadership hasn't been easy. A lot of sacrifices came from this calling. I acknowledge how much of me you must have missed. I didn't have a choice. As I reflect, I don't know what I hated most — the mental, physical and emotional strain of dealing with institutional constraints; the faulty medical treatments for people facing system challenges; or the rift that taking psychiatric and opioid medications caused between us. Actually, I hate the fracture the most. We were living the American Dream. I feared losing it all, so I followed their directions. I was wrong. Nevertheless, I am proud of you both. I have no doubt that God will restore.

To my friend, Keshay J. Williams, you've been a solid support and positive presence in my life. Thank you!

To my cousins, Lavette Minor and Alex Minor, thanks for endless hours on the phone with me, allowing me to laugh and cry while protesting my growth.

Lastly, to Ronald Reagan UCLA, I am thankful for ten years of service. Still, I am concerned for your employees. There is a better way than discrimination.

BIAS and
BURNOUT

"Burnout is nature's way of telling you, you've been going through the motion but your soul has departed; you're a zombie, a member of the walking dead, a sleepwalker. And false optimism is like administrating stimulants to an exhausted nervous system."

— Sam Keen

INTRODUCTION

Stress, Burnout and Disease

Knowing the key physical signs and symptoms of any impending stress-related disease is crucial for gauging where you are in your situation and your recovery. Just as important is knowing the signs of burnout.

First, chronic stress is related to the decision-making process. Fight or flight is your personal bias.

Failure to make an informed, critical decision will lead to burnout. Burnout is the end-stage of chronic stress. Burnout begins when our thoughts fixate on an object of desire. Instead of doing what is necessary, we overthink, avoid, and do anything other than face the challenge. For instance, let's consider a perceived imbalance of power. You want to do something oppositional such as file an administrative complaint of discrimination. Perhaps you wish to confront someone making you feel uncomfortable.

Perhaps you want to refuse management's request to do something that may disadvantage another. Perhaps you wish to blow the whistle on unsafe or unjust business practices. You may fear repercussions. If you were not afraid of being fired or suffering retaliation, you would do what you know is the right thing to do. Such double-mindedness causes moral distress, leading to mental exhaustion, burnout and health disparities.

Instead, you can have health equity. Centers for Disease Control and Prevention (CDC) defines *health equity* as a condition "when everyone has the opportunity to be as healthy as possible."

Racial injustice makes it hard for anyone to own their power. You have to learn how to spiritually fight for justice. You have to know all opposition offer an opportunity to be advantaged. In this book, I'll show you the exact power moves that I used to my advantage — preventing my own health disparities.

Discrimination is a perception issue. To escape the madness of adversity, look inward. Then do exactly what scares you, what challenges you. Do what is true for you. No one else has to agree with you about what is happening to you. Your perceptions are your realities.

Fighting institutional racism is mindboggling. You may think that you are losing your heart and your mind. People may tell you that if you fight back, you risk sabotaging all you have worked hard to achieve. Risk everything. Rather than succumb to feelings of inadequacy, you can become a powerful leader in your job and your life.

Better days will come. There is hope. You are not helpless unless you give away your power. My two-years under psychiatric care due to institutional bias revealed to me the 180-degree difference between the *Diagnostic and Statistical Manual of Mental Disorders* and the Word of God, my guiding principles.

May I suggest that you turn around. Change direction. This is a fight for your life. Don't take flight from responsibility by hiding behind the mask of mental illness.

We face personal health risks by remaining silent about bias issues that cause chronic job stress. Not knowing the rationale for reporting injustice, you may think, "It's not my job to say something," but you are morally liable.

Confronting workplace bias could threaten your job security. Fear and anxiety are natural responses to this risk. When you see the benefits of speaking up for yourself and for equality, then you gain the security and confidence to make a power move that makes a difference.

How we think about ourselves is strongly related to our sense of belonging to a community. Once you join a workplace community, your employer expects you to uphold the community policies. When you're hired, your onboarding process covers organizational, state and federal anti-discrimination and anti-harassment laws to protect the potential victims of age, race, sex or gender bias. These policies are reinforced in your annual reviews. However, your employer likely has not taught you how to apply all their equity policies.

What you are missing is the health equity information crucial for feeling emotionally safe to examine your own prejudices and confront someone else's.

If management fails to treat you equitably, over time, you may turn bitter and cynical. Cynicism can turn you against a career you love. Work that once inspired you to show up and do your very best now burdens you.

Whenever you feel insecure as an employee because of mistreatment, protecting your ability to keep earning an income lies in knowing your personal history, judging your current situation and making a power move.

When you have some semblance of understanding your role in health equity, you can identify the potential health outcomes of action or inaction. Planning becomes simpler. You gain a more precise evaluation of health promotion, putting your own health first.

Without critical decision-making skills (such as those learned in the nursing process and health equity training), essential workers may be subject to the adverse health effects of systemic employment discrimination. When professionals like nurses and other healthcare workers know how to correctly solve complex problems with ease and intelligence, the employer, the employee, health consumers, and taxpayers all benefit.

My solution is a Health Equity Plan, an adaptation of the five-step nursing process, based upon the scientific method: *Assessment, Diagnosis, Planning, Implementation, and Evaluation*. I've modified this process for addressing bias and resolving conflicts leading to burnout.

You can delight in a life free of the inequalities caused by systemic racism. If you are willing, confront racist behavior on your job. To win, you must play on the proverbial chessboard — ready to move, ready to wait, ready to risk. Use your power to protect the most essential piece. You are the king. God's promise is that you can never lose a good thing when you make good decisions.

Knowledge and application together are the keys to wellness. Empowering yourself will improve clinical outcomes. Would you like some help navigating through the murk of discrimination? My life proves it's possible.

I grew up in turmoil. Inimical childhood experiences were my everyday life. I never saw myself as a statistic until I endured institutional racism and sexism in the healthcare system as a registered nurse and as a Black woman with a disability. The control administrators exert unfairly over employees, for me, induced dire thoughts. Discrimination is chronic stress.

I faced great evil in the healthcare system trying to find my way to justice. To be honest, I wanted to kill somebody. I wanted to die. I thought of suicide to escape. When coping with adversity, for humanity's sake, we must learn to conduct business. Letting go of my attachments — to my self-image as a nurse, to my pay and benefits, to my social circle, family, and friends — was critical for me to reach health equity.

Beyond being a nurse, as a healthcare consumer under my employer's managed care plan, I felt coerced by the doctors to take inappropriate medications to deal with job stress. These included steroids, narcotics and antidepressants. Ineffective medical treatments (with little or nothing to do with the racist causes of my job stress) financially benefited Big Pharma and health corporations, even my employer. I was disadvantaged. I was harmed.

I'm not the only one who has suffered from workplace discrimination. According to the U.S. Equal Opportunity Commission, an average of 90,000 people file complaints of discrimination every year. The majority of these filers are African-American women.

I'm not the only one who saw a doctor for job stress and was told to take a prescription to deal with discrimination. I'm very disappointed with the medical industry's treatment plans for job stress produced by bias. We need education before medication to cope with stress.

Introduction

People gave me lots of advice, but no one gave me any solutions that could work for me. No one told me how to help myself. I needed healthcare workplace representation, education, advocacy, and support. Now I'm sharing with you what I have learned from my journey.

May I show you the way to health equity?

"Thus saith the Lord, Stand ye in the ways, and see, and ask for the old paths, where is the good way, and walk therein, and ye shall find rest for your souls. But they said, We will not walk therein."

— Jeremiah 6:16

ONE

Pain and Purpose

Call me Moses! I've always wanted to say that. As a young girl, I was enamored with Harriet Tubman. I felt she and I had many similarities —our vivid dreams, our calling, our career paths, our desire to serve others.

Like me, Harriet was a nurse and an activist who was passionate about civil rights. She's also a Davis. A thirst for freedom awakens hunger deep down in Davis bones. We can't rest without going back to deliver those last few laborers who want freedom from strongholds.

Living in conflict with an employer will change your way of life. For nurses or anyone, such moral distress is a scary, uncertain place. Your image, your faith, your health are all on the line. There is hope in pain, and a purpose. The subtle complexities of *pain* and *purpose* are powerful life-changing motivators, intimately intertwined.

The distress of conflicts with management on the job, uniting pain and purpose, I have found, can bring us into our fullest life potential. Working knowledge of job stress may help us reach our potential in the healthcare system and other industries.

Few healthcare professionals know how to address the pain and purpose that come with the conflict and stress built into the system. Our healthcare workforce is untrained in how to be fully empowered as employees. We all are left vulnerable to victimization, including burnout.

Nobody likes conflict, yet what if your opposition in the workplace is like the story of David and Goliath? Chosen for a great task, do you find your greatness? Do you find you have all you need to slay your giant? First you need to discover and use the tools you already have. Your victory may mean better health, a job promotion, a leadership role, or entrepreneurship.

Healthcare professionals have mental health resources available, yet they are burning out and committing suicide. As healthcare employees, we want workplace solutions that will heal us and not harm us. We want health equity. We want workplace equality.

Too many employees, perhaps yourself, cope with job stress by opting to take psychiatric or opioid medications at their doctors' recommendation. Such treatment plans are not preventing job burnout. When these people become addicted to prescription drugs, lose their jobs and end up in poverty or homeless, society is told they are suffering from untreated or under-treated mental illness. The real problem is not knowing how to handle job stress.

One may say the system failed the burnouts. I say the burnouts failed by not exercising their right to health equity. Knowledge of the causal link between job stress and poor health can prevent employees from becoming corporate and pharmaceutical waste.

There are no safety nets for you if do not put your health first. If you ignore your spirit, what you know inside is true, the resulting hard times are predictable. If you change your mindset, you change your outcome. Why wait for a policy change to save you? This is your chance to slay the Goliath of job discrimination.

The healthcare workforce is shrinking. A 2018 survey of 700,000 physicians by the Physicians Foundation found that 78 percent of the doctors said they "sometimes, often or always" experience feelings of burnout. The study also reported that 46 percent plan to change careers. COVID-19 has intensified these feelings of burnout.

Today and in the pandemic's aftermath, the employees who remain should have access to a health equity nurse skilled in *workplace healthcare equity.* They then would have different outcomes than the millions of burnouts who never received any health equity information.

Before Burnout

Before I tell my story, let's define burnout. Burnout is a state of emotional, physical, and or mental exhaustion. Burnout is caused by moral distress, marked by unhealthy attachments, a fear of loss. Burnout occurs when you feel overwhelmed and drained, unable to meet daily life and work demands. Emotionally, burnout leads to clinical depression. Physically, burnout weakens immunity and induces diseases. Mentally, burnout disrupts cognition. All three states will harm us unless we stop the repetition. All three stress conditions overlap our spiritual responsibilities to heed our conscience, to make the right decisions for society, and to put our own health first

I know all about burnout from my own professional journey as a registered nurse.

I decided to become a nurse in 1996 while working as a medical assistant at a women's health center in Fort Worth, Texas. I admired the warm professionalism and confidence of the nurses. A decade later in Los Angeles, I earned an associates degree. My first real nursing job was as a care partner at the UCLA Santa Monica hospital.

In 2007, upon graduation, the UCLA Center for the Health Sciences recruited me as a critical care registered nurse. I loved being a critical care nurse. I was excellent at it. I could gladly have retired as a critical care nurse. Staffed with the brightest minds, the Medical Intensive

Care Unit (MICU) managed multi-organ system failures for patients transferred to us for the highest tier of care. We did everything possible to save lives. Our teamwork was impressive. We united as professionals into a loving community. We shared fun, laughter, travels, marriages, parties, food, and lasting friendships.

In October 2012, while giving medications to a patient through a naso-gastric tube (goes up the nose and down to the belly), I used a 60cc syringe to push a thick mixture of green bile and medication into my patient's stomach. As I pressed the syringe plunger with the thumb of my right hand, I felt fire shoot from my thumb up my wrist. I repositioned my hand to give my patient back his stomach contents. I then sat down in the alcove, put a cold pack on my sore wrist, and charted my nursing assessment.

The unit charge nurse noticed my cold pack. When I was still using a cold pack a couple days later, my nursing manager told me to file a "doctor's first report" as part of a formal worker's compensation insurance claim.

The doctor in the UCLA occupational health office said flatly, "I don't see any reason for you to be using your thumb at work." I should have asked him to chart that comment, but I was too distracted by his gaze, his look of amazement that a Black person and a woman could do such high-level work. He seemed astonished that I could walk and talk and use my human opposable thumb.

He recommended over-the-counter pain medications, icing my wrist and returning in two or three weeks if I did not feel better. My pain persisted. The occupational doctor referred me to a UCLA sports medicine doctor who was a specialist in hand injuries. To rule out other causes of my pain, she ran a battery of serum tests.

The tests showed that I was borderline positive for antinuclear antibodies with a nucleolar pattern suggesting system lupus erythematosus. My official diagnosis was osteoarthritis of the thumb, de Quervain's tenosynovitis and tennis elbow. I received two weeks paid time off through worker's compensation, steroids to reduce inflammation and a snug wrist brace to wear daily for two weeks.

By the next visit, from muscle atrophy in the brace, I'd lost strength in my wrist, and my shoulder hurt. I told her about this new pain. She dismissed my complaint, saying, "but I thought it was your wrist." All I could do was hope the pain would go away. The pain didn't go away.

My worker's comp physical therapist noticed a limited range of motion in my wrist and an inability to engage the small muscle groups in my right hand. She suspected I had thoracic outlet syndrome and requested authorization for shoulder rehabilitation. UCLA's workman's compensation insurance company, Sedgwick, denied the request.

The UCLA sports medicine doctor then referred me to Dr. Christopher Zahiri, an orthopedic surgeon under contract with Sedgwick. I visited his office in Beverly Hills to seek a full assessment, diagnosis and treatment plan for my injury. Without any explanation beyond saying my original complaint was only for my wrist, he refused to look at my shoulder. His attitude seemed dismissive to me. I felt unheard. I felt invisible.

By now six months have passed. I'm doing "modified duty" not permitted to do direct patient care. Instead, I'm assigned to help train the new nurses on the team.

Soon, they no longer needed me at all. Because I was on modified duty, I was coded differently than the non-injured employees for pay, time and attendance. I wasn't counted in the daily staff census. I could come and go as I pleased, with no nursing duties. I felt unaccountable and segregated from the rest of the team. Afflicted by chronic stress and pain, I felt lost and hopeless.

I felt a lack of healthcare support. Their medical skills were fine, yet cultural bias — structural discrimination in the training of physicians — filtered their treatment of me. They treated me as a high achieving uppity Black woman with no right to complain about a prestigious job they felt I was lucky to get.

In my mind, I saw the people closest to me laugh, skip and hop right over me, going on with their merry lives. I saw myself crawling on the floor, struggling to get somewhere, anywhere other than where I lived in pain.

I needed to be believed. I needed that listening ear. I needed help to lessen my burden. I needed the confidence to cope with employment discrimination. I needed treatment that was for me, not against me. I needed the courage to wait, trusting in my own heart, mind and soul.

A Health Equity Plan

Avoiding the chronic job stress that leads to burnout requires a health equity plan. Similar to having a business plan, you need a reliable road map. A holistic approach to healthcare planning can promote workplace equality. My views are faith-based, yet these core nursing principles work regardless of faith. I'm sharing my insights with the hope that you will empower yourself.

Health equity begins with workplace equity. You are a valuable person. Failure to execute essential skills when conducting business with your employer can potentially leave you vulnerable. Like in any business, you have goals and objectives to consider for growth. Unless you have a practical strategic plan, how can you succeed?

It's hard to be in conflict with your employer. There's so much at risk. Luckily, as a gainful employee, you have a wealth of job benefits to use along the journey.

However, if you do not stand up for yourself in the workplace, the procedure for remedy can be one-sided in favor of the corporation. If you do not take a stand, you are left looking for help after you fall, and there are no safety nets. In real time, you must stand up for your own value. Stand up for the ethical use of workplace policies. "Good faith" efforts to uphold the just rights of staff and management will be honored in any fair court of law.

You may think you have a winnable case, and you get excited about "sticking it to the man." The problem is that many job discrimination claims never get to a judge. Their cases close in arbitration or mediation settlements between attorneys, but plaintiffs seldom find peace.

As one who never wanted to be anything other than a registered nurse, I cry to witness compassion fatigue among great nurses when we genuinely care for others. Seeing profits put before patients, we discuss the issue, but we fear standing up for our rights and risking our pay. Do you feel forced into putting your health on the line to get a paycheck and benefits? Systemic employment discrimination happens in all industries, not just hospitals.

My own professional experiences have convinced me that our corrupt business practices have single-handedly caused America's public health crises, including today's unpreparedness for the COVID-19 pandemic.

A recognized social determinant of health is the effect of bias in workplace policies, disadvantaging vulnerable populations. I feel it is my soul duty to raise up the nursing platform by providing workable equity solutions.

My pain can help you find purpose. No one likes pain. I wish I could tell you there will be no pain. There will be great pain — physical, emotional, mental, and spiritual pain. You may lose faith. You may long for what feels safe, familiar and "normal."

Great rebirth can arise from feeling crushed, under pressure, alone in the abyss. See the dark night of the soul as an incubation period, a butterfly emerging from the cocoon. You are renewed, resistant to burnout.

Workplace health equity is at the center of the process to prevent burnout. Workplace health means more than training employees to ask for help lifting heavy objects. It involves communication and comprehension of the health equity principles that will end health disparities.

Health equity places people before things. A business owner may think a desk has more value than a person. To a nurse, only the person matters. When you put the people first, the venture prospers and the staff thrives.

In our post-pandemic world, the surviving workforce needs to be better prepared at a cellular level to deal with the increased production demands. Many people will be stressed and overwhelmed by the pressure to meet job expectations. Without health equity in our workplaces, our jobs will feel like slavery. Burnout will become widespread.

Our workforce is desperate for better healthcare. Now and in the uncertain years ahead, a top priority is mapping out clear health equity objectives. Holistic health strategies and honest conversations about structural racism can improve clinical outcomes and prevent health disparities. I believe we nurses, and all professionals, need to have the political will to end the adverse health effects of discrimination in our nations. We can do this by adopting the idea of a health equity plan to have open conversations and settle our inequity disputes.

We the People

People are created equal, not created to lose their life, health and wealth by battling corporations. I have evidence proving that gains occur as a result of defying the status quo. Go against the grain if you believe you are not being offered what is right for you. I did this successfully to reach health equity and workplace equality. So can you.

I'm here to remind you that you deserve better. I'm offering an innovative approach from a registered nurse for people who work and want better health.

I believe that our health and wellbeing are our souls' top priority. Will you allow your innate survival skills to drive you towards harmony? In dealing with simple or complex workplace issues, following an equity plan will improve your health outcomes. Since we're dealing with policies of justice and equity, this is spiritual warfare. Any failure means poverty, disease and death.

I personally do not care what name you use for God. I believe Jesus Christ came for us to have life and to have it more abundantly. Regardless of your beliefs, adopt a righteous mindset. I care that you do not lose your life for a false sense of job security.

As a discriminated person with employment rights, you are wise to be wary of professionals telling you that the doctor alone knows what's best for you. This is a false narrative. The doctor's expertise is worth hearing, and so is the nurse's knowledge, but you know what your soul needs. Ask for what you want. Ask what else you can do. All of your conversations with health professionals must empower you, not lower your willingness and ability to defend yourself from inequality. Take responsibility.

We can free our pain for a greater purpose. We do this by our willingness to make informed choices at pivotal turning points. We make the power moves that shift us from painful imbalance to passionate purpose.

The road to health will take the same amount of effort as the road to disease. Which path you take is exclusively your choice. I ask you to prepare yourself for better health and career results. I ask you to get the education you need to pursue your inalienable right to a healthy workplace.

TWO

Power Moves

We can study upstream factors like race and class as social determinants of health. We can name structural racism as a cause of health disparities. However, until we educate people about the role of stress in health, until we provide healthcare support to people coping with institutional discrimination, victimization will continue. The system is powerful and it's hard to change, but we can overcome its attempts to disadvantage us.

We all have a story to tell. Mine is how I went from a tumultuous childhood to a victorious battle with a hospital, the worker's compensation system and psychiatry to serve as a Health Equity Nurse. What is your story?

I have known about "mental illness" my whole life. My beloved mother was diagnosed as paranoid schizophrenic with schizoaffective disorder. My maternal grandmother carried this diagnosis, too. Had my ex-husband lived long enough, my nursing experience says he may have been diagnosed with bipolar manic depression. Instead, at 27 years old, he ended his life by jumping from a thirty-foot bridge while running from the police.

My mental health issues surfaced when I was struggling with the healthcare system after my injury.

I had been on worker's compensation for more than eight months. I saw I was not going to receive an accurate diagnosis for my shoulder. The allotted physical therapy sessions for my wrist were coming to an end. I contacted my worker's compensation case manager at Sedgwick. She refers me to UCLA's disability manager, Mark Briskie, who never reached out me. I could hear papers rustle on his desk as he searched for my file, then he said, "Oh yeah, Glennae Davis. How can I help you?"

I told him that Sedgwick had told me to call, and we scheduled an in-person meeting. At our third meeting, brandishing a pen and a coy smile, Mr. Briskie offered to make all this go away. All I had to do was agree that I am better, and I could return to the medical ICU.

I said, "No, Mr. Briskie. I cannot do that. I am in pain." I'm thinking, I cannot use my hand the same as before, so how can I safely care for vulnerable patients and myself? "I am here to discuss my workplace options as a BSN." (BSN is registered nurse with a bachelor's degree.)

Mr. Briskie called Dr. Zahiri, who set an appointment for me. At that visit, Dr. Zahiri came into the examination room and asked, "Do you want to go back to work?"

"Yes, but I need another position, one without direct patient care, because I'm still in pain."

He released me to return to work, but with permanent weight restrictions of ten pounds and not more than ten minutes of computer work per hour. I was not okay with these restrictions. Ten pounds. Really? I was already doing modified duty, so why render me virtually useless?

He then gave me a "zero percent rating." In California, the permanent disability rating determines the amount of money to be received as compensation for a permanent disability from a job injury or occupational disease. A ten percent rating would have given me 30 weeks of wages. A zero percent rating meant that I had no reduction in my earning capacity, so I was not entitled to *any* compensation for the loss of income from my on-the-job injury.

What made me even more angry is that the weight limit and computer restrictions made me unfit for almost any job unless I got an accommodation, but a zero percent rating meant I was not entitled to an accommodation.

In other words, they said I could go back to work with no record of disability, but the restrictions kept me from working even if I was not in chronic pain. I thought, they could have kissed me before they screwed me!

I had defied the odds of a hostile childhood, earned a college degree and worked for many years as an excellent employee. I had become a homeowner. I was living the American Dream. When I chose to assert my rights, that's when a diagnosis was used to disempower me.

When I was fighting for health equity, I felt despair and confusion. I was afraid of losing my job, and people in my church kept saying, "You better keep that good job." I didn't know how to do what I knew in my soul I needed to do. I needed to have the mind of Christ in coping with a system of discrimination. Fighting racism at the policy level is harder if we fight using the ways of the world.

Instead, I deserved advocacy, support and education to pass this test of faith in God and in myself.

Achieving Health Equity

How can healthcare professional address health equity issues for vulnerable populations when we ourselves are a vulnerable population? Job stress and burnout is causing nurses and doctors to quit or commit suicide. Our plight is made more urgent by the COVID-19 pandemic.

We nurses certainly love the work that we do. We are confident managers of care. Dressed in scrubs, we stride down hospital hallways, stethoscopes hanging from our necks like capes of steel. We save lives. Saving lives is what we do. We don't have jobs; we have callings.

But at what cost? We sacrifice our bodies, our families, our holidays, our futures. Other professionals visit doctors with legitimate complaints of job stress, yet we don't deal well with our own stress. Before we can help our patients, we must be willing to help ourselves first. Let's protect our own lives while coping with job stress.

I recommend that we nurses, the same as all professionals, find an ally for coping with stress. Job stress is difficult to handle because our way of life, our financial resources and sense of belonging are all tied closely to employment. Strategizing with a health equity nurse, who specializes in chronic stress and workplace inequality, can empower us to keep doing the work we love.

With a health equity nurse, we can improve...

- clarity about the causes of our job stress,
- understanding of our risks and opportunities,
- communication between management and staff,
- comprehension of workplace right,
- self-confidence to ask for our rights,
- planning for our power moves.

Whatever grand vision we may have for our future, our story begins with a thought. Health begins with how we think. To walk through discord without giving away your power, it takes positivity, power, guts, and glory. It takes courage to survive stress, to make the breakthrough into liberty and to live life in abundance.

Ten Power Moves

Working as a Health Equity Nurse, I've identified ten *power moves* you can make for your own advancement. I invite you to study these concepts and master the ability to make these moves in your own life.

1. **The Power of Risk** — Take personal risks for the sake of spiritual and worldly and fulfillment.

2. **The Power of Thought** — Trust your innate talent for reflection, judgment, contemplation, and reason.

3. **The Power of Vision** — Vividly imagine the outcome you desire. Allow yourself to feel grateful that it's already real. Gratitude empowers our visions.

4. **The Power to Focus** — Focusing your energy brings forth an inner fire to light your way and inspire you.

5. **The Power to Protect** — Take steps to shield yourself and those you love from harm. Guard your life and preserve your safety, physically and spiritually.

6. **The Power to Ask** — Be willing to inquire, request and interrogate. Ask vital questions and expect an answer. Require a response and claim your right to know.

7. **The Power to Confront** — Exert your natural right to confront your accusers. Insist upon a fair examination and discovery of the truth. Light dispels shadows.

8. **The Power to Pray** — Connect to God, as best you understand God. Plea for help, or affirm that divine help is yours. As for me, I pray in the name of Jesus Christ.

9. *The Power to Wait* — Practice patience. Find your inner stillness. Allow time and space for major events to unfold. Meanwhile, sustain an expectation for a positive outcome. Have patience. Hold faith. Stay the course.

10. *The Power to Breathe* — Where there is breath, there is life. No matter how much we may fear the worst, so long as we can breathe, we can feel hope to do the work of turning our vision into reality. We can let God breathe inspiration into us, communicating divine instructions into our minds.

Using these power moves did three specific things for me. The moves eliminated my own bias, so I made good choices for me, regardless of others' opinions. The moves advanced my career within UCLA, and they saved me from subjection to the system.

You can use these power moves too. When conflict happens, decide what action you will take. The goal is bringing yourself to peace. Whether you believe in Jesus Christ as the author and finisher of faith, God is our infinite source. Take advantage of the gift.

Making power moves builds character. I strive to be an excellent employee. I do exactly what my boss asks of me. However, when a boss requested ethical breaches — that I lie (falsify documents), accept a lie as the truth, cheat (divert organs), or steal (inflate charges) — my moral distress shifted my boss from UCLA to God.

Moral distress happens because we become aware of what's right and true. It is a calling. Not everyone on the job has this awareness. Some have an unconscious bias. I'm talking about bias against African Americans that presumes we lack the knowledge and skills do our jobs, let alone lead the organization.

Black people are keenly aware of the improvements needed in the workplace. Instead of making room for us to grow and contribute, we are stifled and antagonized. The bias will drive us into burnout unless we make power moves that are inclusive and advance us.

What we want is harmony between work and life. With a good work/life balance, we can enjoy a seamless exchange of compensation for a job well done.

I can tell you first-hand the hardest power move is choosing to confront. Confronting requires vulnerably, knowledge of your expectations, and hard conversations. This is how we lead organizations without moral distress. This is how we avoid burnout and create equity.

Make these ten power moves when there is trouble, and the spirit of God will save.

THREE

Chronic Job Stress

Thinking through my situation after being released from worker's comp with permanent restrictions, I was concerned that my modified duties didn't match my job description. Since my annual review was coming up, I asked my unit manager about my job status, "Could I be fired for not meeting expectations?"

He said, "Technically, yes." Then he reassured me that he was in my corner.

I began to study the UCLA disability policies. As a qualified person with a disability, I should have been offered a meaningful position as an accommodation. I was hopeful about continuing my career at UCLA.

In May 2013, a church sister and colleague who works in kidney transplantion informed me about a lung transplant position that will open soon. She told me about what the coordinators do, their perks and high pay. She reminded me that in the ICU I already worked closely with Dr. David Ross, an attending pulmonologist in the MICU and director of the lung transplant department.

I immediately emailed the nurse manager of the lung transplant department, introducing myself and inquiring about the soon-to-be open position.

Later that day, I saw Dr. Ross and said, "I hear there's a position opening up in your department." His eyes glowed in approval as he said, "Yes, I think you would be wonderful for the job."

Later that week, the lung transplant nurse manager called me to report all the good things Dr. Ross had said about me and to offer me an interview. During the interview, she said, "I see what Dr. Ross sees in you." She added that they wanted to hire me but first had to go through the process of announcing the position publicly and interviewing others, but not to worry. The job was mine.

In July, my colleague in kidney transplant forwarded to me a "heads up" email from a co-worker in the lung transplant department that they just had a staff meeting and should make a hiring decision by Friday.

The next day, I received a follow up email from the kidney transplant coordinator that "HR did an exhaustive review of all the candidates' HR files and was moving forward with other candidates."

I emailed UCLA's nurse recruiter to ask if did not get the job because of my modified status. She said, "No."

Later that day, when I saw Dr. Ross in passing, he put his head down and avoided eye contact.

I emailed the nurse manager who interviewed me to ask if she'd made a hiring decision yet. She did not reply. I sent two more emails before I finally got her response: "There must have been some misunderstanding."

I kept receiving a paycheck for showing up five days a week, eight hours a day, and doing nothing. I remained hopeful. I applied for 13 other positions at UCLA. In many instances, I was declined five minutes after applying with a cold note, "Good luck on your future endeavors."

In other instances, I went to interviews where they did not follow the standard job interview procedures and asked questions that indicated they already had prejudicial information about me. I viewed these as fake interviews. I felt humiliated by the apparent pretense.

One interviewer actually said to me, "You act like you deserve a job." Well, as a qualified person with a disability, legally, yes, I did deserve a job.

I felt that I was being discriminated against, so I retained an employment attorney. In September 2013, I filed an administrative complaint of discrimination based on disability with the hospital and the Equal Employment Opportunity Commission (EEOC).

Living under chronic job stress increased my physical and emotional complaints. I wanted to be treated equally, but I was being treated as inferior.

I felt frustrated. I felt institutional constraints were oppressing me. Hospital administrators used their power to disadvantage my way of life, my health and my career just because I have a record of disability.

Their inability to see my ability induced psychological pain. Their bias about my disability made me aware that they saw me as useless and disposable. They saw me as unworthy of being a contributing part of any team.

I knew I was caught between a rock and a hard place. How could I trust the cunning administrators who said, "I am trying to help you," as they impeded the flow of my employee rights in favor of the hospital's financial interest.

Stages of Stress

Failure to eliminate any giant stress challenge can lead to death, disease, low self-esteem and a mediocre life. Giants are unique to each of us. The mental, physiological and emotional reactions are not.

Appreciate that job stress is a perception issue. Start by ruling out the presence of any actual disease. Focus attention on what stresses you. If you identify a conflict between doing your job well and keeping yourself well, that inner conflict will create cognitive dissonance.

Nicolas Cole labels the "Five Stages of Stress" as Fight or Flight, Damage Control, Recovery, Adaptation, and Burnout. He advises knowing which stage you are in.

Physiologically, when we experience stress, activity in the thyroid and adrenal glands increases. We may try to control the stress, but if it continues, the glands will overload, leading to a sense of "burning out."

As stress persists, the body next pumps out far more stress hormones, raising heart rate, increasing blood pressure and decreasing short-term memory, which further increases stress, fear, anxiety, and depression.

The body then adapts to the higher levels of stress. Recovery seems to happen as the stress gets normalized. Mental focus briefly improves

Meanwhile, the physical damage continues. Unless the source of stress is removed, the physiology collapses. Full-fledged burnout results, causing clinical depression and hospitalization for stress-induced diseases.

Our perceptions of stress and burnout are very real. Unmanaged job stress is a valid health concern. Learning to confront job stress head on, in most cases, can remedy the situation, especially when dealing with coworkers or supervisors whom you feel abused to be around.

A moment of private conversation with a nurse trained in health equity can reap a lifetime of emotional rewards that eliminate stress and lead to a better quality of life.

Instead, employees see their doctors, get a diagnosis and then are prescribed antidepressant or anti-anxiety pills to help them tolerate job mistreatment.

If you chose to take a pill, that's fine. Remember that delaying effective decision-making (flight or fight) will cause stress levels to remain high. From this book, you are gaining the knowledge and education you need to protect your health with the backing of a health equity plan.

Work/Life Imbalance

This is why teaching all employees to manage their responses to workplace stress is key to preventing suicides, homicides, workplace mass murders, and domestic violence. In my professional opinion, psychiatric medications are not fit remedies for coping with job stress and related issues. I want to see better healthcare options for coping with the real-life root causes of disease.

In medicine, *acute* and *chronic* are timelines. Acute refers to conditions lasting less than six months. Chronic refers to conditions lasting more than six months. For many, living one day in raw pain may be too long.

Tom Beckman, director of the Health Professionals Program at HeartMath, cites studies going back decades that 60 to 90 percent of all visits to doctors' offices are for stress-related ailments. Some studies assert 75 percent of all physical diseases result from unhealthy emotions.

According to a 2015 study by Paul E Greenberg *et al* in *Journal of Clinical Psychiatry*, "The Economic Burden of Adults With Major Depressive Disorder in the United States," job stress costs companies a fortune.

Expenditures for Major Depressive Disorder (MDD) in 2015 exceeded $210 billion, a big increase from $173 billion in 2005. Almost half (48 percent) of the total are workplace costs, such as absenteeism (workdays missed and "presenteeism" (reduced job productivity from being present at work but not working). About 45 percent of the expenditures are direct medical costs (like outpatient and inpatient services or pharmaceuticals), and these costs are shared by employers, employees, and society as a whole. About five percent of these costs are tied to suicide.

As a healthcare practitioner and healthcare consumer who knew adversity my whole life before experiencing chronic stress from systemic employment discrimination, I deeply resonate with such research. You may find these studies are confirmed by your own experience.

Symptoms of Stress

I wish to share the common signs and symptoms of stress that may lead to burnout, if left unresolved.

Our nation's burnouts become unemployable, drug addicted, violent, homicidal and suicidal. Many of them have or had full-time employment. Have you ever stared at a homeless person and wondered what happened to them? I have, and I talk with them. They confirm how job stress can be devastating.

If you are uncertain about what might be your own stress symptoms, below is a general summary:

Physical — Low energy, headaches, digestive issues (dry mouth, difficulty swallowing, nausea, dyspepsia, diarrhea, constipation, incontinence), muscular problems (tension, aches, pains), pulmonary and coronary issues, (colds, rapid heartbeat), circulatory issues (cold hands or feet), nervous disorders (twitching, tremors, clenched jaw, teeth grinding), tinnitus, infections, loss of libido.

Cognitive — Insomnia, unsettling dreams, constant worry, racing thoughts, unable to focus, illogic, unsound judgment, disorganization, forgetfulness, pessimism.

Emotional — Agitation, frustration, moodiness, lack of control and desperation to assert control, unable to relax, self-doubt, poor self-esteem, avoidance, loneliness, worthlessness, feeling overwhelmed, depression.

Behavioral — Procrastination, irresponsibility, altered appetite (overeating, undereating, bulimia, anorexia), abuse of addictive substances (alcohol, drugs, cigarettes), nervous actions (fidgeting, pacing, nail biting).

This is by no means a comprehensive list, yet I believe this is enough to persuade you about the dangers of stress, specifically job-related stress. If you still need convincing, think about the long-term consequences of unresolved stress in your life. A short list of the problems from long-term or chronic stress includes mental health disturbances like anxiety, personality disorders, deepening depression, and eating disorders like bulimia, anorexia and obesity.

Physical issues include gastrointestinal problems like ulcers, gastritis, colitis, and irritable bowels. More severe risks are cardiovascular disease, heart disease, high blood pressure, arrhythmia, heart attacks, clots, and strokes.

Less dangerous but still vexing problems include acne, eczema, psoriasis, and hair loss. Reproductive and sexual issues are menstrual problems for women, and impotence or premature ejaculation for men, plus lost libido for any gender, which may disrupt or end relationships.

Do you see the big picture that job stress can kill you? Distress endangers your mental and physical health. If you cope with medications instead of eliminating the conflicts causing the stress, this can be life threatening.

When you experience conflict with management that produces acute or chronic stress, you are in the desperate throes of controversy. Nothing else matters but the conflict. You may be too overwhelmed to live your life.

Power is the capacity, ability and willingness to act. Use the power move of thought to identify the source of your agitation. Reflect on the nature of your situation. Judge its seriousness and consequences. If you are being unfairly disadvantaged due to bias, your power move is to protect yourself, future generations and the communities you serve. Make the power move of risk, dare to take Godly action, trusting yourself, knowing you are more valuable than any company bottom line. In time, making these power moves will bring you forth to light.

The solution to job stress is workplace health equity.

FOUR

Confronting Bias

The California state legislature once considered a collective bargaining law for registered nurses based upon a disheartening view of our healthcare system. According to Assembly Bill no. 1201:

> "The institutional force of health care facilities and medical group providers has turned against the interests of patients and health care consumers as a result of the managed care reordering of economic priorities and incentives. As a consequence, licensed direct care registered nurses are the only potentially effective means for assuring the provision of safe health care services for patients."

Does this view of healthcare surprise you? It shouldn't. Like every business with financial goals and stakeholders, healthcare ventures aim to make money. Even nonprofit healthcare organizations require money to keep operating. Modern medical care is expensive to deliver, which means care providers like nurses carry an ethical and fiduciary responsibility to employers and patients alike.

Nurses are a primary resource in healthcare, the same as doctors and support staff, from records clerks to janitors. As a registered nurse, I want to meet my fiduciary responsibilities to provide care in my patients' interest. This is true for all of us in healthcare.

Take my own case. After I filed my EEOC complaint, another position opened in the lung transplant department in November 2013. I felt both excited and puzzled. The job notice gave the address of the liver transplant office, not the lung transplant office doing the hiring.

I showed the job notice to the MICU nurse manager and pointed out another oddity. The announcement said an applicant must be able to "lift 25 lbs and handle heavy volumes of data entry." The nurse manager gasped and said, "That does not belong there!"

Was this requirement inserted into the job description specifically to discourage me from applying? Was I being excluded by discriminatory language because of my job disability or my EEOC complaint?

By then I'd been dealing with corporate attorneys, corporate doctors, middle and upper management, the union and chief nursing executives, but I was getting nowhere.

Were they all colluded against my health equity efforts? Because of my physical condition and the worker's compensation decision, I feared losing my license. After I had worked so hard to become a nurse, I was exhausted by the obstacles I encountered to keep doing what I loved.

So, I emailed Dr. David Feinberg, President of Ronald Reagan UCLA Medical Center. I blew the whistle.

The Effects of Bias

There are real-consequences to implicit and explicit bias based on gender, race, age, religion, disability, or other factors. In the workplace, bias shows up when rejecting qualified candidates for employment, promotion and accommodation even though, on paper, they meet all the requisites. To conform with the real or perceived bias of management, hiring managers often miss a chance to employ experienced and dedicated talent.

A groundbreaking study by the Los Angeles Homeless Services Authority, released in 2019, found that biased policies are the primary cause of racial disparities, including employment and health disparities.

I believe that when managers and employees learn to interpret policy without bias, when we stop fighting what feels natural and apply inner knowledge, then we will prevent systemic discrimination, victimization and burnout. We will increase the profit for people and hospitals.

Dr. Cartwright Do Wrong

There's a strong correlation between chronic job stress and major depressive disorders. We can see the dangers of misunderstanding this connection by looking at how it was misconstrued to justify slavery in America.

Let me take you back to a time before the Civil War and introduce Dr. Samuel A. Cartwright, a physician in Mississippi and Louisiana. To explain why slaves ran away from their masters, he published a biased 1851 paper in which he invented a disease called, "Drapetomania." He hypothesized that a mental disorder or madness akin to alienation caused Africans to flee captivity. Ignoring the natural human desire for freedom, he said slaves ran away when they felt isolated from the plantation community. His cure was treating the slaves as children. Pacify them. He never questioned the institution of slavery.

The essence of institutional racism has not changed, only the outer form. Today we are employees, sometimes paid quite well. Now doctors use pharmaceuticals to repress our desire for freedom. Enslavement transcends race.

If you are employed, how much freedom will you assert? Are you willing to confront bias at the policy level? Are you willing to risk your paycheck, benefits and social status for true health? If you want to protect yourself from the negative health effects of bias, if you want worklife harmony, what are you willing to do?

Begin by recognizing you want the freedom to pursue happiness and self-fulfillment. Begin by acknowledging that unresolved conflicts with management cause chronic job stress. Recognize the struggle is between your rights and their profits, which can be exhausting for you.

Burnout occurs when we are dependent on a system that has no life to give us. A corporation, by definition, is an artificial person. Let us not die feeding it our life. Make power moves. We can stand up for our rights. When we do not, we are nothing more than slaves.

You Need a Health Ally

I agree with Dr. Cartwright that our desire for freedom alienates us from those who exploit us. We do become detached if we feel used. I disagree with how our institutions treat valid complaints of bias as a mental illness.

We really need navigation, not medication. I wanted to be told that I was doing the right thing by standing up for myself. No one showed me a good way forward.

I lacked a health equity nurse. I lacked a guide showing me how to fight workplace battles spiritually.

Are you in a similar situation? Perhaps you have come far in life. Maybe you have a home and amazing children who depend on you. Maybe you have professional knowledge and a license to protect. Do you need an ally? Get one who has the insider secrets to overcome racism.

Do you know you have the right to defend yourself — in real time — from being disadvantaged? Once you file complaints about violations like a hostile work environment or retaliation for whistleblowing, coping with this added stress poses fresh challenges. You need reliable guidance to handle the spikes of stress hormones.

If you think complaining about workplace bias will be an easy payday, think again. Filing lawsuits are costly. You risk living the rest of your life with regret. Your best power move is finding a health equity expert to guide you with a health equity plan. You need an ally.

Above all, be clear about the outcome you want. Use your power move to breathe. Rest from action or toil. Affirm yourself. Express good about yourself. Manifest your future self. Connect to your soul.

Connect to God, your greatest ally.

The love of God is simple, perfect and restorative.

FIVE

Disease or Wellness?

I blew the whistle! I wrote a letter to the head of the hospital about what had been happening to me. Let me condense my lengthy letter:

> Dear David Feinburg, MD
> I am writing to you to make you aware of the three adverse job actions against me... I am now a "Qualified individual with a disability" [who] was repeatedly declined positions that I qualified for, as well as my applications being rejected at HR.... It is my belief that [the lung transplant nurse manager] found out about my modified status and chose another applicant. I continued to apply to different transplant coordinator positions, and I believe that the nurse recruiter blackballed me from getting interviews or sabotaged those pro-

spects. Mark Briskie [the disability manager] has been no assistance in the matter. His position is that I should be satisfied with coming to UCLA while remaining on pay status. I am a qualified individual with a disability and demand a meaningful job, one that enriches my life and the lives of others.... I need help, and I would like a meeting with everyone involved in mishandling my disability and violations of my rights.

Thank you,
Glennae Davis

Years of discrimination, blatant disrespect and denial of my workplace rights, including lost job opportunities, had made me sick. My hair was falling out. My skin had erupted with severe acne and sun sensitivity that left dark blotches on my face. My joints were hot and swollen. My ocular pressure and blood pressure were both too high. I had gained 30 pounds. I was at risk of a systemic lupus diagnosis. And my arm still was in chronic pain.

I was dealing with at least seven administrators with unconscious bias who were dictating my rights. I was done being a pawn on their chess board. I decided to make a power move. I wrote a letter to Dr. Feinberg.

I exerted bold and professional behavior with the expectation to gain the fullness of my rights. I wanted wellness. I wanted wholeness. Protecting my territory has never been an issue for me. I'm a gangsta from the Jungle, but I never had no street hustle. I never sold anything. I only knew how to be employed. I only knew I had to stand up for myself in the face of scary opposition.

When it came time to assert my rights at the hospital, I remembered where I came from and who I am.

Within a week after sending my letter, I received a call from the big boss of the disability office. She offered me two positions. The first position was in the obstetrics and gynecology clinic. I'd worked in OB/GYN as a medical assistant, and I did not wish to go back, so I declined that offer. The other job was as an inpatient lung transplant coordinator — the exact position I wanted!

I accepted the job as a transplant coordinator. To this day, I don't know why they put weight and keyboarding requirements into the job description. I barely used the computer for charting (data entry). I didn't carry anything heavier than my cup of coffee. I was happy, at first, but soon, not so much.

What stayed in my mind was a warning from the disability manager when she offered the job. She said, "Don't start no trouble." I didn't start anything, but trouble found me. Shortly after I began working, as I was walking down a hallway with a colleague, both of us laughing, I saw the chief nursing officer coming toward me. As she walked past, she rolled her eyes at me!

That hallway incident heralded what was to come. I did not believe that I had done anything wrong, but I felt ashamed about the way I got my job. My using the law for leverage had upset people.

Hostile Work Environment

I settled into my new job orientation process, meeting coworkers and learning the culture. Human resources sent a friendly note congratulating me on my promotion.

A few days later, my case manager at the EEOC called me at work. Now that I had the desired job, she asked, would I drop the charge of discrimination? I felt disbelief. The audacity! I reminded her about the denial of jobs, the fake interviews, and ignored request for mediation.

"But now you have a job," she said.

I responded by talking about other staff experiencing job discrimination. They didn't seem willing to speak up for themselves, so my complaint was as much for their benefit as mine.

The EEOC manager, a Black woman, replied, "Don't worry about them. Worry about yourself."

"They are me." I took a breath. "So, you can tell UCLA that I said no. My complaint stands."

After two years of fighting the worker's compensation system and hospital administration for equality, I was not about to let the EEOC dismiss my case.

Once my orientation ended, I devoted myself to being the only in-patient lung transplant coordinator. I worked closely with my transplant team, educating my transplant patients and their families about life after transplant. I felt my work mattered. I felt spiritually nourished.

Then I began to notice my white peers were watching my every move. I began to feel they were breathing down my neck like an overseer. They showed up unannounced at my educational sessions, scrutinizing my work, offering unsolicited advice, as if I didn't know what I was doing. I ignored them at first, and then I started asserting my competence. I found out later that they'd run to the boss to complain about the way I set boundaries.

I saw that my white peers had one-on-one meetings with our nurse manager, but I did not. In fact, they attended my supposedly private meetings with her. Next, I saw that I was excluded from office meetings in which my work assignments were discussed without me. I'd find out later about duty changes affecting me.

On the surface, the workplace environment appeared calm and pleasant. Still, I could not shake the feeling that something was brewing behind the scenes. I felt violence in myself. I felt vulnerable, psychotic, delusional and paranoid — and I could not prove anything. The more I talked to others about what I thought was happening, the crazier I sounded.

My first night on call was a total disaster. My job that night was coordinating both heart and lung transplants. I specifically asked the nurse manager if there was anything I should know before going on call. She said, "No, you'll do fine." Well, I did not do fine. I did not have the phone number for hospital admissions. I did not have the pre-op schedule to prepare patients properly. I did not have the organ procurement workflow for getting organs from donors to patients. I did not know that I was supposed to be sure the procurement team was fed. The chief surgeon got angry at me for not following the expected procedures by contacting him before the organ arrived.

The next workday, I brought to my nurse manager's attention my concerns about my painfully obvious lack of specific knowledge for coordinating the organ transplants. She was dismissive and said "Oh, didn't I give you this training manual?" She handed me 17 pages of material, and had me sign a receipt for it.

"You know we haven't done this before," I said, as I handed back the receipt.

"Oh, I guess we haven't," she said with a big smile on her face. I believe now this white woman had been directed to withhold this crucial information from me, setting me up to fail. I believe the hospital risked the lives of the patients in our community, and the department's reputation, to disrupt my career and my life. Retaliation.

The hostility increased my physical pain, withdrew my zeal for life and depressed me. I no longer knew what I needed or wanted. I could not validate my experience. I could not find my way to liberty.

I was caught between being a liberated Black employee and a dependent descendent of slaves. I struggled with cognitive dissonance. I was looking for consistency, but my only constants were my ongoing arm pain, my job qualifications as an RN and my inalienable civil rights.

I knew something had to change, but I didn't know what. I emailed my nurse manager, asking for a meeting to discuss my pain. She declined, saying, "I appreciate what it must have taken for you to ask for help, but I have a program to run and other employees to consider. You understand, I have business decisions to make."

I then discovered another meeting was held about me but without me being present. A part of staff reorganizing, I was assigned added responsibility for coordinating heart transplants as well as lung transplants, an impossible double duty for even an able-bodied person. The two teams actually met separately at the same time on the same day. How could I be in two places at once?

Instead of getting help to assure safe patient care, I was given a heavier workload that disadvantaged me. This struck me as retaliation, another microaggression because I am Black and because of my EEOC charge.

At that point, I would rather have died than reach out to Mr. Briskie about my unrelenting pain, my feelings of discrimination and my unreasonable workload. I did not want to start any trouble, as I'd been warned against doing. At the same time, I could not picture myself doing both jobs at once while trying to restore my health; but if I don't, how could I pay my bills? How much more injustice could I take? I was out of options.

Self Advocacy

Your response to bias in the workplace directly affects your health. You can ride the turbulent waves instead of being shipwrecked. You can restore your mental, spiritual, physical, and financial health if you seek health equity.

You may think fighting for justice shouldn't be that hard. People simply should not discriminate. We should just follow the law. Sadly, that's not always the reality. We each are accountable for advancing our own lives through our choices. Make good decisions, get good consequences. Make poor decisions, get bad consequences. The choice is ours. We all have freedom of choice.

I wish that achieving work-life balance was as easy as creating laws that make other people stop disadvantaging us. However, no law can prevent you from disadvantaging yourself. A janitor and hospital president are both able to use workplace policy to protect their interests.

Organizational culture directly determines employees' willingness to follow organizational policies. I have heard healthcare leaders say, "My hands are tied." I have seen pain on the faces of nurse administrators wanting to do right by me but stopped by upper management. Be willing to do what's right for yourself and the company, which means using anti-discriminations laws without bias.

When it comes to institutional constraints, your hands are never tied. Stand up for yourself boldly, professionally, and the perceived chains fall off immediately.

Our nation's workforce is facing a health crisis that goes far beyond the high cost of medical care or the recent pandemic. Without workplace healthcare equity, worker addictions, preventable diseases, poverty and burnout will continue to increase.

Racial bias, such as white supremacy, can be defined as doing what you feel benefits your ethnic group while disadvantaging another. There is one Creator to serve. No matter what name you use for the divine, serve God with all that you are. We need your gifts and talents to develop equitable systems with healing leadership.

Nurse Advocacy

Since I became a nurse, working with patients of all ages, I've found that empowering them to make informed decisions and speak up for themselves is the core of nursing. For instance, a patient diagnosed with liver failure was not an ideal candidate for a transplant. His only option was remaining in the ICU, receiving ineffective care.

The morning we met, he had been laying in a hospital bed for five days deciding whether to die now by natural causes or die later by complications from futile medical interventions. He was sad because his requests to die in dignity were not being respected by the staff. He told me, "They are not listening to me."

We chatted during his morning assessment. He asked, "Will you tell them to let me die?" I glanced over at his beautiful wife, her eyes swollen from crying. Hearing his request, she began to wail.

Using a nickname he'd given me, he pleaded in his Mexican accent, "Black Beauty, I want to get in my truck, lean back and see the sky one last time. If I don't make it home to my bed, so what? I'll die on the street like a dog. I've lived a beautiful life, made love to my beautiful wife, raised four beautiful children. It's time for me to go to the clouds. I am alright with that." We connected.

Upon researching his chart, I learned that a few days earlier, because the patient didn't agree with the plan of care prescribed, the medicine team consulted psychiatry, which diagnosed him with clinical depression. Psychiatry then started him on antidepressants, suggesting that he take time to think about his decision to die.

I observed the patient was lucid and clear about what he wanted. So, I held his medications and called a team meeting. Psychiatry, the medicine team and I discussed our findings. My patient was placed on end-of-life care. By the end of my shift, he'd passed away with his family at his bedside, thanking me for defending his wishes.

Extended medical care for the sake of research is a noble cause, when a patient chooses to participate. Such study can benefit future generations. Nurses are advocates for our patients. The nursing side of the medicine team advocates for the whole person, what we call wellness. The medical side focuses mainly on injury and disease.

If you are a nurse, when advocating for your patient and yourself, reject any negative thoughts that you are not enough. The going may get rough. You need to calmly sail the troubled waters between anti-discrimination laws, workplace policy and healthcare regulations.

I advise using the *power moves*. For example, if facing bias at work, use the power move to ask vital questions. Use the power of thought to understand your situation. Use the power of vision to get clear about what you want. You *can* use your personal power and benefit.

"America's health care system is neither healthy, caring, nor a system."
— Walter Cronkite

SIX

Conflicted Decisions

I was encountering a hostile work environment, and no one could relate to my need to be obedient to God, not even the church. No one showed me how to let go of my stress, let go of my attachments to money and status. No one taught me how to handle my situation sanely, how to be true to my soul and keep my job.

Americans have a bad habit of quitting a race before the end. A few people stay the course, but for some odd reason, many think they're not supposed to suffer, so they give up before reaching the finish line.

If you do not know that the kingdom of God is within you, that passion leads to destiny, then you need wisdom. Discerning the difference between a door being closed and your divine authority to move any mountain by grateful faith will lead to an abundant life. Bypass the obstacle. Keep advancing. This was true in my case.

I regretted entering the worker's compensation system. I missed my days working in MICU. I wanted to go back to feeling joy with my career and life in balance. Now my life was in turmoil. I could not trust my employer's intent. I did not always feel hope for my future.

One day, an East Indian female co-worker decided she no longer wanted to be in the transplant department. The work no longer served her need. She applied for a new position doing direct patient care. She interviewed and was gone. That broke my heart. I could not be like her. I could not decide for myself what was best for me. Her transfer showed I was in a trap. Was my ceiling from being Black or disabled or from filing a discrimination complaint?

I felt confused. I was doing well financially, better than I could have dreamed. I was a homeowner. I'd gone from making $13.01 per hour as a medical assistant to $150,000 per year base salary, plus up to $20,000 per month stipend for being on call, plus a handsome benefits package. It all added up to a comfortable life — economically.

I'd gone from gang banging to a seat at the table. Every morning, I discussed the allocation of organs with world-renowned pulmonologist, immunologist, cardio-thoracic surgeons, and professors of medicine. I never once felt as if I did not belong in those meetings. I established a good rapport with all the physicians on the transplant team. I had earned respect as a competent professional.

What was missing? The administration could not let go of their bias against me, nor leave me free to do my job. They stifled me. I could not be myself. I could not progress. I could not ask for what I needed like others on my level. Bias limited me. Lack of diversity invalidated my perspective. Biased practices antagonized me. Stress flooded me. Fear paralyzed me. I was drowning.

Many times and in many ways I was told, "Let it go." "Move on." "You should just be happy with what you have. You've come so far. Don't risk losing it all." I didn't feel heard. I didn't care about any of those things. I was in a tug-of-war over life and death. I lost my strength. I became a shell of my former self. I lost my heart, my courage and my brain. I felt like the characters in *The Wiz*. Following the yellow brick road, I'm off to see the Wizard.

Consider Your Soul

I went to work every day, educating and empowering my patients to take control of their health. I want them to know the side effects of their medications. I want them to learn how to set healthy boundaries that will give them their best chance of survival. I'm telling people to do what I'm unwilling to do for myself. I am a hypocrite.

I'm still in pain and still afraid to tell Mr. Briskie about it. I am afraid to open that can of worms. I am afraid to start trouble and deal with his hostility.

Reality hit me in summer 2014 when Robin William committed suicide. I heard media commentary that he always wore a smile, making others laugh while he must have been dying inside. This sounded like me.

My sojourn led to a sorcerer psychiatrist. She was an average-sized white woman with sandy brown hair who wore Bohemian clothing. I sat in a dark chocolate-brown leather chair. Its wood arms seemed strangely protecting. That moment was the safest I'd felt in a long time.

"Tell me," she asked. "Why are you here?

"I don't want to be here!" I cried, "Have you ever been some place you don't want to be?"

"Where is here?"

"Here, with you, scared. I feel caught somewhere between subjection and liberation."

I sobbed out two years' worth of hurt, disappointment, and frustration. I told her the story of my injury, my worker's comp claim, my EEOC claim, my physical pain, my attempts to get a job accommodation, my sense of discrimination, how I experienced it every day. She shifted around in her chair as I spoke, taking notes.

At the end of her 45-minute hour, she diagnosed me with Major Clinical Depression. She prescribed Cymbalta, taken daily by mouth, PO QD. To keep a Delusional Disorder diagnosis off my record, I told her that I'd retained an employment attorney. She put down her pen.

I saw my psychiatrist once a week. I took the antidepressant every day. The medication claims to offer adjunct pain relief specific for muscle pain. I had hope.

The prescription drugs Cymbalta and Ultram were a double whammy. The psychiatrist prescribed Cymbalta, an antidepressant. The pain doctor had prescribed Ultram, a synthetic opioid. No one noticed the contraindications. The combination almost ended my life and career.

Nobody questioned my medications' behavioral side effects. While on both these medications, for the first time in my life, I became out of control, impulsive, scared and doubtful. I said and did things out of character for me. My voice changed. My children said they didn't know me.

I wanted to give in to my darkest impulses. Some days I wanted to die. I had more than enough prescriptions and sample meds to commit suicide. My life looked perfect on the outside. My inside was in shambles. I felt isolated and trapped. I thought, how can God be the answer, when this is so painful? How could God bring me to a place where I've acheived so much and yet expect me to risk it all?

The situation was bigger than me. I chose to trust that if I did this hard thing — confront bias, risk my job, risk my way of life, and break free of institutional restraints — that God would provide. My only responsibility was to honor the truth of my experiences. Anything less would be devaluing myself.

Over that summer, the antidepressant's side effects became increasingly adverse. A metallic taste tainted my favorite foods and drinks. I had chronic constipation. I could not sleep. Each morning was a mournful continuation of the day before. The Monday grind lasted all week. Images of revenge overtook me. I literally had to get down on my knees to pray for each of my enemies by name.

Every step I took demanded energy I did not have the reserves to give. Arriving at my patient's bedside in a profuse sweat, I must have looked like hell. Cymbalta brain zaps punished me whenever I tried to form a thought, so I kept my composure. My flat affect gave the impression all is well. Nothing about me was well.

Due to the antidepressant I was emotionally dead. I grew numb and despondent. I could walk into a moving 18-wheeler and feel nothing. I felt alone. Misunderstood. I'd fallen into an abyss. The only way I knew I was alive was that my arm still hurt.

I knew there had to be a better way to live. I chose to focus on my relationship with God and put health first.

In the fall, I said to my psychiatrist, "I don't want to take these medications anymore." I told her that the meds were not fit for human consumption.

"Oh, Glennae," she said with sympathy. "Employees take psychiatric medications all the time to tolerate company politics. If you stop, what else will you do?"

I sat in silence, thinking what else could I do? I am in so much pain. I cannot breathe.

She broke the silence, "Glennae, it's been six weeks. You are not tolerating the medication, and you should not be still upset about the company making business decisions. You should try Electroconvulsive Therapy."

I was taken aback. "Who still does ECT?"

"UCLA Neuropsychiatry department has as an area. We can do it there."

"What are the side effects?"

She replied, "A little memory loss."

I said, "I'll think about it."

I realized that she wanted to help me forget about my oppression by inducing a seizure in my oppressor's house. She wanted to shock my brain happy.

I was adamant about not wanting to use Cymbalta any more. For me to detox safely, the psychiatrist wrote a medical order that I could not work while detoxing.

During our subsequent weekly visits, my psychiatrist continued trying to put me on other antidepressant drugs as well as anti-psychotic medications.

She said that if I didn't take prescription medications, or else do medical interventions, my disability insurance company may not believe me, and may not pay me. She advised taking a drug at night, cutting it in half or taking it every other day, but I *must* start taking meds.

In my mind, I heard the Scripture, "O taste and see that the LORD is good: blessed is the man that trusteth in him. O fear the LORD, ye his saints: for there is no want to them that fear him." I have one God to serve.

Detoxing

Big Pharma has warning labels on antidepressants about side effects like odd or sudden changes in behaviors, such as aggression or suicidal ideation. In my professional opinion psych medications contribute to poverty, homelessness, domestic violence, and even homicide.

I was in a state of dis-ease without any evidence of a diagnosable disease. I was burning out. I questioned myself. Was I really sick? Was I making it all up? If I was, for what purpose? Why sabotage my life? What would I gain? The meds kept me from doing the introspective shadow work that I needed to do to get my life back on track.

I asked my psychiatrist about natural alternatives for clinical depression. Without hesitation, she recommended that I do high-endurance cardio exercises and eat whole foods. She also recommended N-Acetylcysteine (NAC), known to help the neurotransmitters in the brain.

NAC immediately lifted my mental fog, which some call a "veil of depression." Over time, the NAC supplement increased my body's oxygen absorption, which improved my exercise stamina and facilitated healing.

Cymbalta, had not stopped my pain, and taking ibuprofen did not relax my muscles. I felt like I was pulling a load too heavy for my body. My buttocks pulled in toward my core. My shoulders lifted toward my ears. My head tilted slightly backward. The stress caused me to clamp shut my jaw, cracking four molars in my mouth. For relief, I started ingesting hemp oil, which helped.

I next received a letter from the psychiatrist saying that Mr. Briskie at UCLA's disability office had requested a copy of her psychiatric notes about me. She wanted my permission to release these notes to him. This pissed me off. He'd used his authority as a UCLA official to request private mental health records not directly related to my worker's compensation. I felt violated. I declined.

Mr. Briskie then made an appointment for me to see a forensic psychiatrist. What? He wants my mental health evaluated by someone who can testify in a legal proceeding? Why? I concluded UCLA's attorneys were trying to build a case against broken down little ol' me.

I declined the invitation.

"Natural forces within us are the true healers of disease."
— Hippocrates

SEVEN

Depressed or Oppressed?

I tried to go back to work. My options were returning to work as if I had no disability, or else asking for an accommodation. I was done being a coward.

I chose to seek an accommodation. In Fall 2014, Mr. Briskie called to say, "Don't report to work." He said that UCLA would pay my full salary while I engaged in what the EEOC describes as an "Interactive Process."

> While an individual with a disability may request a change due to a medical condition, this request does not necessarily mean that the employer is required to provide the change. A request for reasonable accommodation is the first step in an informal, interactive process between the individual and the employer. In some instances, before addressing the merits of the accommodation request, the em-

ployer needs to determine if the individual's medical condition meets the ADA definition of "disability," a prerequisite for the individual to be entitled to a reasonable accommodation.

In brief, to get an accommodation under the Americans with Disabilities Act, I needed an ADA-defined disability, and I had to ask for a *reasonable* accommodation.

The Interactive Process

I had a record of disability-related work restrictions. I could not lift more than ten pounds, nor use a keyboard normally. These restrictions were not acknowledged in my new job description as lung transplant coordinator. Were they deliberately ignoring my disability?

My whole life was interrupted by the injury. I still had unresolved "activities of daily living" issues caused by my workplace injury, which left me in chronic pain. I could barely drive to work, my neck and shoulder and side hurt so badly when turning the steering wheel. Some days, I could not turn the ignition key with my weak and twisted dominant hand, so I had to use the other hand.

At work, I felt the injury most when I had to pick up and carry a load of medications from the pharmacy, or when I had to twist open pill bottles to help patients learn to identify their medications. I felt pain when trying to handwrite patient education notes. I felt depleted from walking the half mile from my office to the hospital for patient visits. I was injured working for UCLA. I'm not yet healed. That injury was interfering with me doing the new job at UCLA I'd fought so hard to get. My days were more taxing than colleagues because I carried a burden of bias.

I'd asked for a reasonable accommodation from UCLA, as the law allows, but UCLA resisted my request. After ten years of loyal service, my needs were ignored.

The accommodation I wanted was simple — rearrange my work schedule. At that point, I could not take a shower and make food on the same day. I asked to take Mondays or Fridays off. A long weekend would give an extra day of rest and recovery before starting my workweek. I offered to work longer hours. I'd still get my job done.

To recover from my injury, I needed to prioritize my health. I needed time to heal. I had used up my worker's comp allotment for physical therapy. Given my exhaustion, an additional day off would let me hire a physical therapist to do rehab work. An extra day of rest and recovery would let me begin strengthening bonds with my young adult children (psychiatric medication had damaged our relationships). I needed the support of my family.

I also needed the support of my company. Instead, the director of transplants and Mr. Briskie created a different job for me, gave it a fancy title and offered it to me. I would be the only "discharge transplant coordinator." Just one catch: I would work every weekend and have Wednesdays and Thursdays off. I'd have to work on weekends when I'd have no staff available, and I'd be home on those days when my busy children were not available.

This was the opposite of what I requested! This made no sense to me. Transplant doctors did not write discharge orders for patients' release on weekends. The transplant pharmacist and the transplant case manager did not work on weekends. What exactly would I be doing all weekend with no patients going home? I'd be wasting precious time. I'd be isolated at work on the weekends and alone at home on weekdays. I'd be out of the office on the busiest days of the week. I'd be unable to contribute as part of a team. None of that was a reasonable accommodation.

This interactive process went on for eight months. The absurdity and hostility I faced were humiliating, degrading and traumatizing. I saw discrimination in action.

Bias was pervasive. During the interactive process, for instance, I was docketed for a job interview in the post-anesthesia care unit. I was told to go. I met with two white nurse managers who were openly gay. At a time when same-sex marriage was being legalized, these two gay people displayed no empathy for my civil rights as a Black woman with a disability. There was no compassion. Their dismissive attitudes exposed how white privilege had kept me from maintaining a successful career.

The Ultimatum

Hospital administrators pressured me to come back to work as the in-patient heart and lung transplant coordinator, but without an accommodation. They wanted me to do the same double duty that had prompted me to quit using antidepressants and taking time off to detox. They gave me one last chance to come back to work by a certain date, or else they would have to replace me.

I thought about what would happen if I got fired. How could I go back to work injured and still in pain? How could I find another nursing job without lying about my situation? What would I say to future employers about why I no longer worked at UCLA, the best in the west?

Feeling fear at the risk of loss, I called my employment attorney and said, "I am going back to work.

"Have they accommodated you?

"No."

"Glennae, returning to work without an accommodation would be a great mistake!" The EEOC complaint gave me a right to sue. "I've got the charging papers right here," she said. "I am going to file. We are going to sue UCLA for workplace discrimination."

I told her to move forward with filing the suit.

I made the power move called "Wait." While I waited, I began to write. My notes turned into a book, *Yet Here I Stand: My Journey from Bondage to Liberty.*

Throughout this journey, many people and friends, out of love, called me unreasonable. They told me that I would lose, that UCLA is too big to fight and win. I almost believed them. This was never a fight over material things, but a spiritual fight over principles and policies.

The core problem was white supremacy and systemic employment discrimination. UCLA's attempts to dismantle me showed that I'd struck a nerve. I was the one who felt the pain from their bias against me for the color of my skin, my disability and my righteous temerity in standing up for myself in the face of adversity.

Let me repeat that chronic job stress is not normal. When you risk burning out from stress, you need to go beyond treating the symptoms of spiking hormones and address the root causes of your distress.

If that cause is job discrimination, although standing up for yourself will increase your stress levels short-term, in the long term, you will save your life.

Perhaps you have heard enough science talk, statistical data interpretation and opinions from health experts who have not experienced discrimination. Their assumptions about what you need will likely miss the mark for where you want to go. Has such advice ended the health effects of discrimination? We need deep systemic reform.

EIGHT

Justice

Harriet Tubman said, "There are two things I've got a right to, and these are Death or Liberty – one or the other I mean to have. No one will take me back alive; I shall fight for my liberty, and when the time has come for me to go, the Lord will let them kill me."

She died an old woman.

I felt the same way as Aunty Harriet did. I still do.

My one regret during the journey is that I didn't relax and rethink the impact of job stress. I didn't want to die from burnout! I wanted to survive. I did so by discovering how to assert my rights and fuck the status quo.

Most burnouts happen because employees want to avoid conflict. They believe in mistaken science, or they are too afraid to take a stand. Instead, nurses can help the people end burnout from bias. Make the power move to health equity by investing in health equity training.

Regardless of your job situation, you deserve the help from a healthcare practitioner who understands job stress and the adverse effects of bias. I lacked a health advocate on my journey, so I learned how to advocate for myself. I learned my equity lessons the hard way.

Fighting for Justice

My childhood psychological traumas led to low self-esteem and low self-worth. I accepted less because I didn't know I could have more. Not speaking up for myself left me with meager crumbs. To change my life, I decided to become self-sufficient.

During the 1980's crack epidemic in Los Angeles, my neighborhood was rife with drug abuse and crime. I lived in the Bloods' territory, Black P Stones (BPS). I never sold or used narcotics, but gang bangers were my schoolmates, neighbors and friends.

I got involved in the Drug Abuse Resistance Education (D.A.R.E.) initiative of the Los Angeles Police Department and the Los Angeles Unified School District. I served as a volunteer in the Southwest LAPD office. I wore a Junior Police uniform, which I was told to take off before going home, so I didn't put myself or my family in danger.

I loved law enforcement. I thought it would be an awesome career for someone like me. In 2001, my brother and I applied to become police officers. I saw this as a rewarding way to pay for nursing school. My brother and I took LAPD's entry exam on the same day. We both passed. I trained at the Elysian Park facility near Dodgers Stadium, hired a running coach and passed the physical ability test. I was excited. I was going to be The Law.

In the end, I was disqualified because of my cultural background. Since I was born and raised in a gang hood, I was judged unacceptable. I was denied an opportunity to enforce the law based solely on bias. I was angry!

In early 2013, after my injury, while I was working on modified duty with my job discrimination case pending at the EEOC, I heard the news about Christopher Dorner. A Navy veteran and a Los Angeles police officer outraged at the racism he faced as a Black man, Dorner eluded a manhunt as he shot at police and civilians across southern California, killing four and wounding three others. In his manifesto, he described himself as "a man who has lost complete faith in the system."

I did not condone his methods, but I empathized with his anger. He tried to do what I did, confront the reality of institutional racism. Like me, he became marked and vulnerable after taking a stand. Like me, he wanted his truth heard and his experiences of bias validated. Like me, he was ignored. Unlike me, he chose the route of revenge to change the system. I chose the mind of Christ to win the war against injustice.

On reflection, I see many similarities between being a registered nurse and a police officer. The most significant is *servant leadership* — customer service at its finest.

Reality Bites

Throughout the interactive process in 2015, while I sought an accommodation, I kept seeing my psychiatrist. I cried to her about every blow UCLA dealt me. She would suggest a new medication. I would recite scripture. She would tell me the insurance company may not believe me. I would say God will provide.

She said I was having a test of faith like Job. In a way I was, but I saw it more like I was having a Jesus Christ moment, bearing a heavy cross. I was going to be crucified. The question was: Would I *really* be resurrected?

Knowing how tenacious I can be, people concerned for my wellbeing said I should give up my fight and go back to work. They all wondered what else would I do.

In July 2015, I reached the deadline for going back to work without an accommodation. Unwilling to fall into the pitfalls UCLA laid out for me, I filed for unemployment, stating I was fired for disability. UCLA did not contest my statement and honored my claim.

I wasted no time calling my lawyer to share the news. She said that since UCLA did not contest my unemployment claim, they now could not be compelled to disclose in discovery the documents or data that would support my charge of discrimination. This meant I had little or no chance of prevailing in court. She dropped my case.

A tragedy and a comedy. I was unsure which was which. I laughed. I cried. An overwhelming sense of peace comforted me as tears of sorrow turned to tears of joy. My blood pressure dropped 110/78.

Immediately after I was fired, I filed an EEOC claim against UCLA for wrongful termination. Soon I decided against it and withdrew the claim. Instead, I would focus all my shattered life energies on becoming whole.

After I was fired, I kept seeing my psychiatrist. As she saw my strength and hope renewed, one day she asked a pointed question, "Glennae, are you depressed?"

She was perplexed by how life was new and better for me. I did not fit the old American Psychiatric Association diagnosis for Major Clinical Depression nor the latest DSM-5 diagnosis of Major Depressive Disorder.

I did not fit her medical models. I took Cymbalta only a short time. I never did ECT. She wondered how I could be healed on my own. I just smiled and said nothing.

My recovery caused a reckoning for her. I believe she no longer trusted her prior judgments about me. My joy baffled her. She leaned back in her recliner chair, let out a gasp of bewilderment, and threw her notes up in the air. The papers fluttered down. This was our last session.

History Repeats

Slavery is America's problem. Early stockholders in the African slave trade sold stolen humans as property to plantation owners. They bought and sold Black laborers for profit. Many corporations today act like southern plantations. When they buy and sell companies, they buy and sell the employees as part of the deal.

I felt like livestock, a commodity traded between my employer, the EEOC, and the insurance companies. It's all a corporate game. They treated me like a pawn on a chess board, sacrificed at will. I was expected to obey my masters' biased rules despite my moral distress.

Am I going too far comparing nurses to slaves?

About 3.8 million registered nurses work in the USA. Between the years 1525 and 1866, according to the Trans-Atlantic Slave Trade Database, 388,000 living African slaves arrived on American shores. That slave count was a mere tenth of the count for registered nurses.

Nurses are trusted and respected professionals, but we face discrimination in our jobs. Bias is most evident if we are Black or a person of color. *Minority Nursing* reports that about 90 percent of all nurses are white, and 90 percent are female. Just under 10 percent of RNs are Black or African American, about 8 percent are Asian; five percent are Hispanic or Latino; and about 0.4 percent are Native American or Alaskan Native.

The problem with this ethnic imbalance is not white people being in the majority. The problem is the evil spirit of white supremacy. Too many white people fear losing their precious white privilege.

We are not our ancestors. Under slavery, my ancestors had no rights, let alone any privilege, but white people today still use privilege to dominate Black people.

We all have *equal rights* under the law, this includes healthcare. A threat to health justice anywhere is a threat to health equity everywhere.

Hope is the evidence of things not seen. Carrying that spirit of hope, nurses need to discern the health effects of discrimination on the job. We must address the bias we encounter at work. The alternative is all nurses becoming the same as African Americans — disrespected, invisible, unheard, and prone to civil unrest.

We nurses are vital gatekeepers to health and wellness. Let us start a conversation among ourselves about how to heal our profession. Let us speak up to protect ourselves and our patients from bad bias. Let us share our nursing knowledge, so our patients heal themselves.

A Trillion Dollar Table

Everyone can benefit from health care delivery. One of those to be advantaged could be you. To reach health equity, take a seat at the U.S. healthcare table.

Centers for Medicare and Medicaid Services (CMS) published a 2020 report on national healthcare spending. Including the $800 billion for Medicare, national health spending is projected to surpass $4.01 trillion in 2020, reaching $6.19 trillion by 2028. America's spending for healthcare will outstrip the Gross Domestic Product (all the economic transactions in the nation).

A major source of economic loss is the tremendous waste of fiscal and human resources expended in fighting discrimination and retaliation complaints, such as mine. I observed upper management's top-down approaches to protecting the bottom line. High production demands on the staff, when influenced by bias, actually interferes with employees' productivity. I am a living example. Because I was not given an accommodation, UCLA lost me, and their patients lost the value of my love for them.

The pressure of keeping employees from speaking out about inequality places stress on the entire organization. The pressure to put profits before people causes fiscal leaks like stress leaves, high turnover rates and lawsuits.

My vision is that our nation will use this moment of pandemic and civil unrest to invest in education and social reforms that uproot systemic bias and prejudice. A rebirth of our justice, economic and healthcare systems will produce equity, respect and justice in our institutions and the communities they serve.

One way to reduce healthcare costs is health equity training for all executives and staff. The emphasis will be on bias and workplace stress to prevent burnout. Ideally, the training is mandatory for all hospitals.

Disease caused by stress costs organizations more than wellness. With the right tools and know-how, our work-force can enjoy restorative rest, creativity and renewed health. With the right systems and process in place, there will be enough money on the table for everyone's gifts and talents to be well compensated. All we have to do is be professional, bold and take a stand for health.

Recovery and Renewal

I entered a time of rest. Every morning, mourning doves would wake me up by scratching the roof above my bedroom. When I went downstairs to my office to write, the doves would perch on the windowsill. This went on for weeks. One day, I mentioned the birds to my son and said God is confirming I've entered into peace. Once I got the message, the doves flew away and never returned.

I was unconscious of time. Each day felt like Saturday. I was amazed by the stillness of life. I was amazed at my creative outpouring of songs and poems and insights. Everything I wanted was there. Living in this state of grace, I could have stayed in retreat for the rest of my days, but I finally felt ready to come back into the world.

In the year after I was fired, I used up my six months of unemployment benefits and withdrew $30,000 from my retirement plan. I was down to $1,500 in November 2016 when I found a fitting new job as a registered nurse at Children's Hospital Los Angeles (CHLA).

My wrist remained twisted and weak. I barely passed strength tests, but I was not in chronic pain. I no longer needed an accommodation — although they asked.

I got into the swing of working again, full-time and on call. After so many years of oppressive rule at UCLA, the playful, heart-centered culture of CHLA thrilled me. The diversity of the staff and relaxed atmosphere fostered a balance in the art and science of nursing. We sang and danced with patients. We wore crazy costumes to work. The children loved it! We nourished those receiving our care. I remembered my abiding love for nursing.

I remembered my calling.

A lifetime of discrimination had prepared me for my vocation. By becoming a health equity nurse, I teach what I learned from confronting bias.

I began working with clients who wanted help. For example, a transgender male faced active discrimination. A millennial worked more hours than she was getting paid. Both suffered severe stress. They gained clarity on their situations and greater confidence to make the power move *to confront* bias in themselves and their bosses.

Working with clients helped me to see the value of seeking expert advice to cope with job stress. In facing systemic racism at UCLA, I lacked a health equity expert. Had I not at least invested in professional advice, I would have forfeited my rights and returned to work enslaved. Potentially, I could have died from my chronic stress.

In the end, my pain led me to find my life purpose. You deserve a health equity expert who's been where you are now, who can help you turn your pain into purpose. You need an equity expert to help you make the power move of claiming freedom and justice in your life. You need expert help to deal with the biased policies.

My Black Life Matters

Despite my education level, social standing or income, my Black life did not matter to "The Man." I followed the doctors' and administrators' advice for coping with chronic job stress caused by systemic bias. Their scientific methods were heavily flawed and almost destroyed me.

Biased thinking may fool us into feeling our hands are tied. In truth, our hands are never tied. We *can* effectively oppose corruption, if we choose. Be good, reap good. Be corrupt, reap evil. Choose the good. Learn to be fearless in pursuing justice. Know that the calamities we see in our communities are from harmful policy decisions. We can do something about it. We can have hope.

Biased thinking may fool us into passivity. We may think our equality and rights are just going to be handed to us. In truth, our natural rights always exist, waiting for us to claim when we hear the calling of our souls.

In terms of mental health, biased thinking may fool us into believing any depressive disorder can be cured by prescription medications. If you have job stress that puts you at risk of burnout, then nothing else in life can matter until you handle your business. You alone are liable.

I accepted responsibility for my life when I realized that I was seeking wholeness from an employer with a bias toward me. I was trying to get from them the acceptance I was not giving to myself. I was looking to be saved from growing. Each time I went to a biased authority figure for a solution, I was left in a worse condition. I finally understood the universal process of growth. I realized that our awareness of systemic discrimination is actually a gift of spiritual discernment.

The Black Lives Matter movement in 2020 produced sustained mass protests in response to police killings of unarmed Black citizens. Despite a pandemic, tens of thousands of diverse people across America and around the world risked infection to demand the end of racism.

Until those affected by discrimination know practical steps for advancement, what I call health equity, I'm afraid the movement will make no lasting impact on bigotry. Unless we create both a social and psychological change, American life will go back to how it has always been — separate and unequal with clear disparities.

Using the ten power moves is how I achieved health equity. How will you? Not putting your health first leads to disease, poverty and death. Eliminating chronic job stress is your most important act of self-love.

This is my highest worship.

"Not by might, nor by power, but by my spirit,
saith the LORD of hosts"
— Zechariah 4:6

About the Author

Glennae E. Davis, BSN, RN, is the CEO of Rx for Life, LLC, a health equity consultancy and education company. She holds a Bachelor of Science in Nursing from the University of Texas at Arlington. Her 16 years of experience as a registered nurse includes the pain clinic at Cedar-Sinai Hospital in Los Angeles, critical care and lung transplant coordination at Ronald Reagan UCLA Health and the Heart Institute at Children's Hospital Los Angeles. Glennae is a poet and the author of *Yet Here I Stand*: *My Journey from Bondage to Liberty.* Applying the gospel to overcome systemic racism within institutions, she writes to share personal and professional insights on health equity.

"We are going to emancipate ourselves from mental slavery because whilst others might free the body, none but ourselves can free the mind."

— Marcus Garvey

Appendices

"Just do right. Right may not be expedient, it may not be profitable, but it will satisfy your soul."

— Maya Angelou

Rx For Life

I am a health equity expert, not an activist. I am about the business of health and wealth. RX for Life, LLC, is a preventive healthcare consultancy and education company with a focus on employment health equity.

TRAININGS:

• **Health Equity Plan** — An 8-week group course that takes an unbiased look at your discrimination complaints and helps you develop an effective legal plan of action.

• **Escape the Madness** —A group class to build your confidence, communication skills, and comprehension for dealing with the causes of chronic job stress

• **Live Well** — A group class that provides healthcare consumers with workplace health care education

BOOKS:

- *Yet Here I Stand: My Journey from Bondage to Liberty.* A memoir of my adverse childhood and later victory over employment discrimination.

- *Bias and Burnout: 10 Power Moves for Healthcare Workplace Equity.*

VIDEO BLOG:

- **Amazing Doers:** Interviews with remarkable people telling their life stories and sharing their views on health at Youtube.com/Naesvision

Warmest regards,
Glennae E. Davis, RN
CEO, RX for Life, LLC.

References

Add Heart FacilitatorTM Program. (2020). Retrieved from https://www.heartmath.org/training/add-heart-facilitator/?bvstate=pg:2/ct:r

Cole, N. (2017). The 5 stages of stress (It's important to know which one you're in). Retrieved from https://inc.com/nicolas-cole/the-5-stages-of-stress-its-important-to-know-which-one-youre-in.html

Greenberg, P. E., Fournier, A.-A., Sisitsky, T., Pike, C. T., & Kessler, R. C. (2015). The economic burden of adults with major depressive disorder in the United States (2005 and 2010). The Journal of Clinical Psychiatry, 76(2), 155–162. https://doi.org/10.4088/JCP.14m09298

Mayers II, B. E. (2014). "Drapetomania" Rebellion, defiance and free black insanity in the Antebellum United States. University of California. Retrieved from https://escholarship.org/content/qt9dc055h5/qt9dc055h5.pdf?t=nk49cg

Merritt Hawkins. (2018). 2018 Survey of America's physicians practice patterns & perspectives. Retrieved from https://physiciansfoundation.org/wp-content/uploads/2018/09/physicians-survey-results-final-2018.pdf

Minority Nurse. (2020). Nursing statistics. Retrieved from https://minoritynurse.com/nursing-statistics/

The American Institute of Stress. (2020). America's #1 health problem. Retrieved from https://stress.org/americas-1-health-problem

The Los Angeles Homeless Services Authority. (2019). Groundbreaking report on black people and homelessness released. Retrieved from https://lahsa.org/news?article=514-groundbreaking-report-on-black-people-and-homelessness-released

Voyages. (2020). The Trans-Atlantic slave trade database. Retrieved from https://archive.slavevoyages.org/

Notes

Bias and Burnout

Notes

Bias and Burnout

Notes

*Of all the forms of inequality,
injustice in health is the most
shocking and inhumane.*

— Martin Luther King, Jr.

Made in the USA
Monee, IL
12 September 2020

42326351R00069